"'I remember...becoming one of the machines,' Shannon Arntfield
writes in her steely debut collection, an exploration of the brutal
sides of medicine and motherhood, where trauma conspires to short-
circuit the present. *Python Love* is a compassionate lament for living
in a body that says 'no.'"

    —MONICA KIDD, author of *Chance Encounters with Wild Animals*

"*Python Love* holds its lines in isolation—granules of memory spent at
the intersections of birth and death, childhood abuse, and moments
of healing. Vulnerable and investigative, this book quietly seeks to
find meaning in the difficult moments while unflinchingly refusing
to look away."

    —CHRISTINE MCNAIR, author of *Toxemia*

Python Love

Python Love

**Shannon
Arntfield**

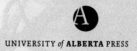

UNIVERSITY *of* **ALBERTA** PRESS

Published by

University of Alberta Press
1-16 Rutherford Library South
11204 89 Avenue NW
Edmonton, Alberta, Canada T6G 2J4
amiskwaciwâskahikan | Treaty 6 |
Métis Territory
ualbertapress.ca | uapress@ualberta.ca

LIBRARY AND ARCHIVES CANADA
CATALOGUING IN PUBLICATION

Title: Python love / Shannon Arntfield.
Names: Arntfield, Shannon, author.
Series: Robert Kroetsch series.
Description: Series statement: Robert Kroetsch
    series
Identifiers: Canadiana (print) 20240481895 |
    Canadiana (ebook) 20240481917 |
    ISBN 9781772127959 (softcover) |
    ISBN 9781772128116 (PDF) |
    ISBN 9781772128109 (EPUB)
Classification: LCC PS8601.R6487 P98 2025 |
    DDC C811/.6—dc23

First edition, first printing, 2025.
First printed and bound in Canada by
Houghton Boston Printers, Saskatoon,
Saskatchewan.
Editing and proofreading by Jim Johnstone.

A volume in the Robert Kroetsch Series.

University of Alberta Press is committed to
protecting our natural environment. As part
of our efforts, this book is printed on Enviro
Paper: it contains 100% post-consumer
recycled fibres and is acid- and chlorine-free.

GPSR: Easy Access System Europe |
Mustamäe tee 50, 10621 Tallinn, Estonia |
gpsr.requests@easproject.com

University of Alberta Press gratefully
acknowledges the support received for its
publishing program from the Government of
Canada, the Canada Council for the Arts, and
the Government of Alberta through the Alberta
Media Fund.

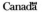

Python Love is dedicated to the mentors who guided me, and the patients who invited me into this journey of lovesuffering.

A special remembrance is made to the mothers and babies whose stories are partially represented here, including Katie and Skip from the DeJong family, and Peri and Jack from the Deacon family.

Contents

Arguing with No One

She was already dying when I was summoned,
when the labour started, attached to machines
the baby was taxing. I remember arguing
with no one—no family, no attending present—
I remember doubling back, carrying forceps,
becoming one of the machines, metallic
heaving head fixed between, no suture lines
to guide us, our only compass the beeping
that rose with every contraction, that crashed on
a shore I wasn't sure she'd reach. Machines
machinating both of us, blind and mute
with fear, our throats constricted, conscripted
not to cry out until I got it out, that ball of flesh,
macerated, silent. The gonging stopped.

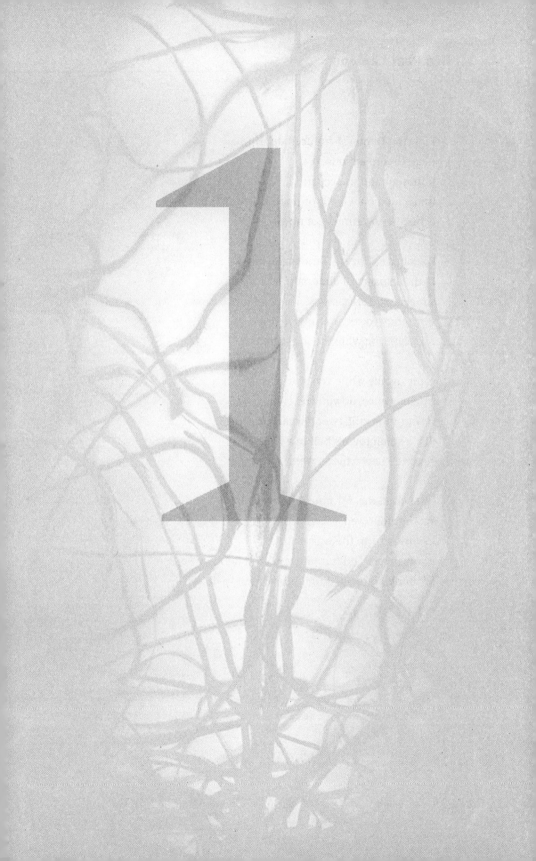

Bed Rest Lament

Fighting Demerol-induced delirium,
no access to anyone,
impotent and unaccepting,
undecided on who to protect—me or the baby—
echoed every time I got no say.

Eyes open, frozen. Dark snake inside.
Python spasm of abdomen
squeezing, contractions,
were they yours or mine? A plea
to escape, he whipped in that place

came awake while you were inside me,
Amelia Grace, do you feel it
resounding still, twenty years later,
like a small town's bell in a fire?
No one knew where I went,

least of all me, for nine long months,
six that followed, when I couldn't
get away from the wasteland
of my pelvis. Did it injure you? Did he?
My body, trapped, didn't know what to do.

Python Love

Coils, thick and writhing,
seek and seal our bodies

in the dark, pulsing
as you grow from spiral

arteries to patent ductus,
fused sinew and umbilicus

between us. An intricate
invasion of blood and brawn,

dual hearts in sync,
immersed beyond emersion.

The Books Said

to wrap you tight babies love being swaddled but you fought for
nine months so no big surprise that blankets were useless / never
use a rocking chair for sleep because one must start as they wish
to continue but you come for hugs when you want them and your
favorite chair is our swing / to not pick you up or hold you when
you cry if training to sleep which I wasn't supposed to start till 6
months but you woke up every hour for three nights in a row and
I couldn't keep going / I couldn't reward you so I cried too couldn't
help you found your fingers that night and didn't lose them till you
decided, fingers in your mouth, soft blankie on your face, and it
was over, just like that.

Tidal Pools with My Mother

Green anemones wave. I poke at their centres,
watch them clench
unfurl;

hermit crabs scuttle swirly brown houses;
bright orange starfish
stick

unmovable blue-black mussels; spines of purple
urchins, my uncertain
finger;

her smile, beckoning me: *a whole universe
hidden*, she let me in,
wide-eyed

on barnacled rock, skin red and indented, knees
aching she revealed her
sense of wonder,

preserved. Far enough away from the dark ocean,
my pressing questions
that smash

on jagged rock. Here, among the shallows,
she keeps me, waves of pins and needle
water, numb feet.

Permeable Membrane

Bodymind   a sieve
for pastpresent

I can't tell who
is touching

me   am I five   forty?
I don't like this

keep my eyes open
send my husband

to my limbic sys
-tem can't pre-

dict the static when
the signals cross

my body channels
the other station makes

me feel so little I am
sick to my stomach

On the Pacific Coast with My Father

Bleached driftwood, sea foam,
rotting fish on rocky beach.
Searching for sunburned kelp—
bulbs that *pop*, hopeful stamping.

Seagulls screaming, picking fights.
Bald eagle in a blown bare tree.
Humpback whale way off shore:
see?   see it there?!   see?

Grey rain sideways down my face.
Waking up at 4am
disoriented and nauseous,
diesel and fish guts on the dock.

Skipping stones on quiet days,
smooth round flat ones
in my hand. Watching his bounce
so much farther, with pride.

Hand in Hand, We Brought Back the Ground

1.

In fall, in workman's gloves,
mother gathered while we scattered
a rainbow of leaves. My sister covered me
in cool earthy kisses as I squealed.

2.

I was so small
on my way to school
and the wind so windy
it blew me from my feet.

3.

I tripped full tilt
skidding arms and legs
in the dress I was wearing
for relatives we escaped.
My sister carried me
all the way back, gravel buried deep
in my skin, pocking her small hands.

Maze Masquerading as a Mangrove Forest

Waving walls split with light
repeating, we turn, turn,

knocking stalks talking, six
feet up. Snap one off

make a flute for your giant.
Air currents brush husks

into parchment wind chimes
I heard in Fan Tan Alley.

Sheaves of yellowed leaves
curl like dry hands.

A purple spider of legs
plunges to the ground

from the base of every plant;
stellate struts radiate—

an axel's bent spokes
gird and guard each sky-

ward birth fourteen feet up:
twenty-two leaves, three ears

of corn, 800 kernels,
each one a seed eaten

or planted. Adventitial
roots brace you in the mud,

brace you in the mud,
brace you in the mud.

The Woman Beneath the Sheet

I am too close to her body,
stiff on plastic sheets.
Eighty-six years old with
pink toenail polish.

My black rubber apron shiny with fat.

Our binder of instructions
flecked with dried up
human detritus
describes bodily functions:

how smooth muscled vagina
makes rhythmic contractions.

My classmate groans,
crown cocked back, puts his hand
on my shoulder, thrusts his pelvis
and wrecks it. He wrecks it.

Blue and Pink Bottles Representing Children

The training was mandatory, you said, black and white
footage of dismembered babies in buckets.
I can't forget that girl I helped who couldn't spell,
dotted her i's with hearts. I was still worried
about abortions then, volunteering to will young
women being thrown from their houses
not to follow through on survival instincts. You cried
a lot, caring for those *Jesus asks us to remember*.
We collected money every year, coins dropped
into blue and pink baby bottles representing children.
Fundraising got us nowhere: out of date pee-sticks
and pamphlets, the basement's cold damp,
the sneering pastor upstairs nicknamed 'the birth canal'
because you painted the hallways pink
to look more inviting. I never did mail you the letter,
what I learned: accident and chance
the sole reason I was not the pregnant girl in the chair.

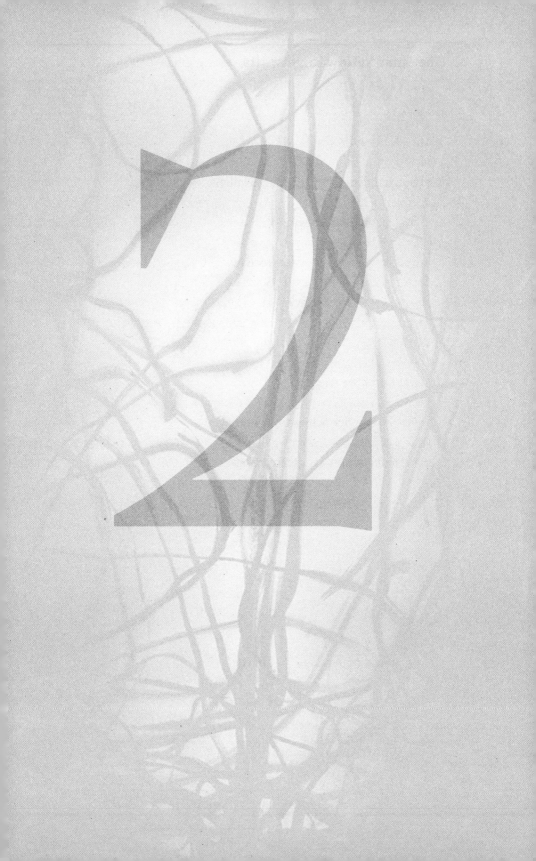

The Same Yellow Tiled Walls

1.

Two pregnant staff   the only available

    help, our due dates

           twothreefive

       weeks shy of—

irrelevant now. We tried to hide

          our bellies from your eyes,

     ballooning   green gowns

       wrapped loosely

          hope hanging.

Your baby

     silent, unmoving.   Infected,

         a virus

contracted while working

2.

inside   the same yellow tiled walls

          you stare   now, silent, unblinking.

We had words   but no reason.

          Offered   a chance to go home

gather your senses

                    had been hijacked

                    by that frozen picture

that black room,

that black screen.

3.

Good stuff happened

all the time—

watching them open their eyes

that very first moment,

shielding the light,

your hand, cupped over forehead;

random meals

together at the nurses station,

crockpot lasagna   uniforms laughing;

dads using t-shirts for Kleenex;

rare midnight coffee-runs;

leaning against the chair back

when it was quiet.

4.

I pull the Gore-Tex   gown down around

        the body inside my body,

            urge

        the body inside yours—

It's time now, let's push.

5.

Came home in the morning,

heaving on the doorframe.

Watched my son breathing,

his chest moving

6.

I wash the long, old fashioned way,

                    yellow-brown iodine

        acerbic viscosity

brush   scrub   squeeze   rub

nail beds   creases   folds   lines

        digit to elbow, both sides, rinse

            scalded, cleansed, start again

        five solid minutes I stretch

to six

in wait,

in supplication.

7.

Given unto us

a purple prayer shawl,

shoal,

shore we washed up on,

coughing,

sand in our hair and

eyebrows.

8.

Writing you later

     on lined stationary—

three little birds, redyellowblue

         perched, each page

an offering—

     his body as you bathed him.

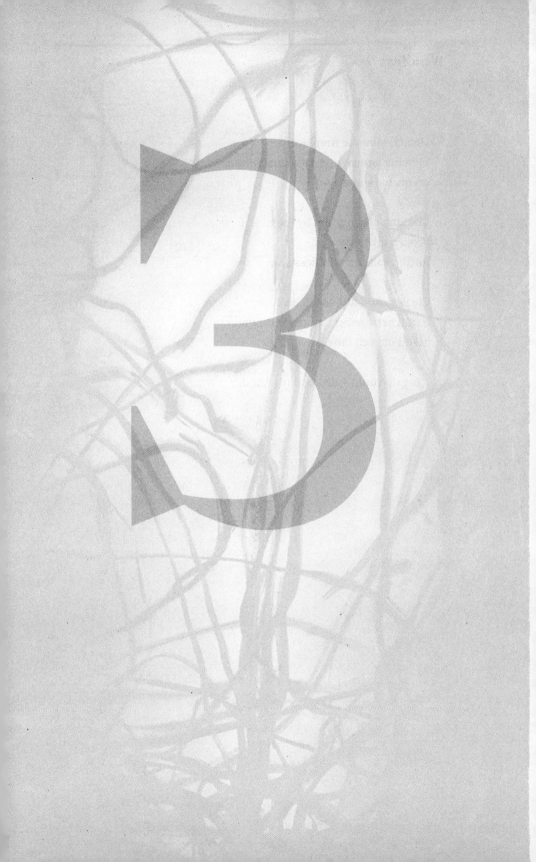

Windless Sea

Head inside the fireplace,
blowing smoke up basement chimney
on his back at 2 a.m.

Couldn't climb stairs by then,
broken alveoli
luffing sails on windless sea.

Clear plastic tubing snaked
a trail between cigarettes and lighter,
green oxygen tank.

His grip could still crush my hand.

Child's Play

I didn't understand
why my friend
didn't want to play
with Barbie and Ken
like I did. Set up

the house, the room
and the bed, strip off
their clothes
and press plastic
pelvis to pelvis.

But I knew from her silence
I'd done the wrong thing.

Clues

When they made her take off her coat
belt sweater shoes
she couldn't say no.

When she caught him in the bathroom,
hands on top of stall,
she couldn't let it go.

When friends took her dancing
and drinking, stares
gripped her ate her burrowed in.

When a man gestured to his hard-on,
said 'I'd like more of you'
and the other waitress giggled.

When a professor explained why some
people don't remember childhood
the lecture hall shrank, quiet and small.

When marriage meant sex—
fingers brushed her blankly.
She made the grocery list.

Car Wash

He drove a shitty little two-door
white Datsun hatchback
with blue and yellow decals,
a fake spoiler on the back.

On Saturdays, I would wash it
while he eyed me
from our stoop, legs splayed out
with his oxygen tank

tripoding elbows braced
on bent knees, puffing
after his walk up the drive.
He pointed out spots I missed

with my dripping, mustard sponge,
paid five bucks to watch
my body and the soap
move in looping sudsy arcs.

Reckoning

Young and strong
erection walking
toward me in a dream

woke me on his birthday,
frozen, long after
his body had gone to ground.

Last to know what he did
to my mother,
to his wife, to his son

first to hear the pus in his lungs,
I'd written him a letter
about God's mercy and grace

the grandsons he could meet,
the burden he might release
if he'd admit he was wrong and believe

he was loved.
The bitterest man I knew
died seeing angels

standing for him, at the foot of his bed.
Thank God
he died

before my mind exhumed
his grip around my ankle,
wild panting in my face.

Get Away

Screaming in the stairwell,
my daughter—

her arms furious   clinging
        pulling on
my body, resisting

transported me

                  I couldn't get him off
                  I couldn't get away

and I ripped her off my leg,
hissing

pushed her

             freeze

                  frame

             freeze

she didn't fall
        but I ran

to get help,
her face pressed
tight against my chest.

Swamp Wading

She told me she could see
the other side of the swamp

      where stinking air pulled
      my body through my nose

all was obscured from my vision
there, in my therapists' office—

      figurines, sand-trays,
      carved caverns
      lit with flares—

I was wading, chest high in slime.

Hyperventilating, chin lifted,
waiting to slip, lose

      my footing
      in a sinkhole, inhaling
      putrefaction.

Cattails waved,
my hand
waving too, too far
to grab

      until she sat down,
      her and my husband
      reached out,

my sister helped
carry, hand over hand
lifted me.

Tickle Attack

He said it wouldn't
feel so bad

if I just stopped
fighting

my instincts
and let him.

There on the mat
in the kitchen.

Jackknifing fingers
splitting my ribs.

A python's grip
my wrist remembered.

A sound—not laughter—
tried to escape.

When My Daughter Turned Eight

my body revolted
in clinics on stretchers online on toilets
expunging, expounding
sudden pain in my gut.

I'd never had problems before, I said.

Then my sister informed me
I wasn't five on that trip.
Look at her eyes.
My child, the same age,

would know what was happening.

God

      carried me

covered in shit

         to her banquet

table. Never

      said I had to.

Never rushed.

      Never pushed.

Gave me dreams

         full of water.

      Stayed with me,

weeping;

         weeping

she washed me.

      Darkness stored

between my legs

         my face

released to her

     light. Beloved

          she called me

     with love she

called me clean.

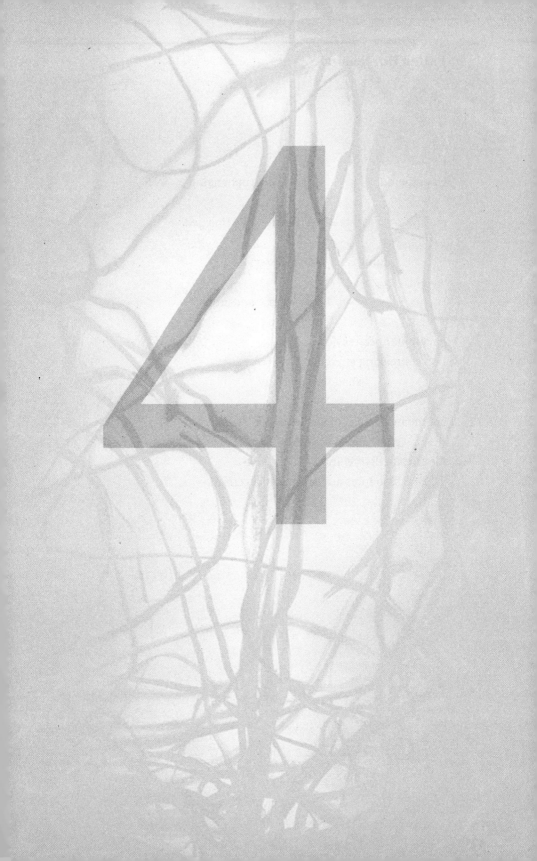

Fallen Horseman

1.

Unprepared   her arm hanging

        thready IV the midwife finagled

   waiting   *come faster*

         lightsandsirens

navy-blue spectres
    streaking stretcher
      shadowed hallway

her moans instead of answers,
    pain? allergies? medical past?
the anesthetist, yelling
      bloodpressureheartrateoxygensats—

2.

Body   full of baby   swept

          from stretcher   to steel

cutting her   clothes off   laying

          skin bare   dumping the prep—

the whole bottle   brown rivulets streaming

          belly to floor   we ripped

                    open everything sterile

          shouted orders   staccato

the silence as we cut

                    my gasp when we saw

          the head

                    floating

it shouldn't be there, it shouldn't be there.

3.

    Blood   casca-
                ding off the
      table
                    her body
   a bottomless

       bathtub

    my whole arm red;

the uterus, dangling   a fallen horseman,

   one foot still in the stirrup.

4.

Folding flaccid parts

are not a whole,

what was split fit

back does not make it better.

Threads of purple suture we used to

put her back together,

back together,

together.

5.

Three days she kept the baby—

       a boy—

              bundled beside her

cold.

                        Like I was blindfolded

                         in a house I knew

                    all the furniture moved—

6.

Thirty seconds to decipher

what was wrong?

why she lay, bluelipped

and

shivering.

7.

Retinal imprint:

apartment, silent

galley kitchen: cream

table I never ate at; single

green armchair, thick textbooks

stacked against it. But my bed, my bed

called like a loon

smudging twilight

stuffed between

slanting walls

that little shed dormer,

puffy red duvet

I had to climb in from the foot end,

happy stripped sheets framed by

the window let in too much light

when I slept, my work life regurgitated,

blood-filled dreams

descending in the daytime.

8.

Hand banging into body walls

knocking shapes I didn't recognize

elbow deep, groping

the space had changed

stop!

An animal, writhing

legs clenched and

arching the small of her back

high off the table.

9.

               Bewildered

         arms
                    pushed at mine

emerging
            white

                    blob of

         holy fuck

I pulled her ovary out

                    she's going to d-
                              ie

                    in fro-
                              nt

                         of
         me
                         a-
                         orta
              pum-
                    p-
ing

              told

         me no

ti-

me

ex-

plai-

n

hole in womb

baby's birth blew

open abdomen

Shouting, we flew.

10.

You caught me

in the hallway, stuck me

in the quiet room.

Sat with me

as you had with the m

-other.

Didn't try to

make it better.

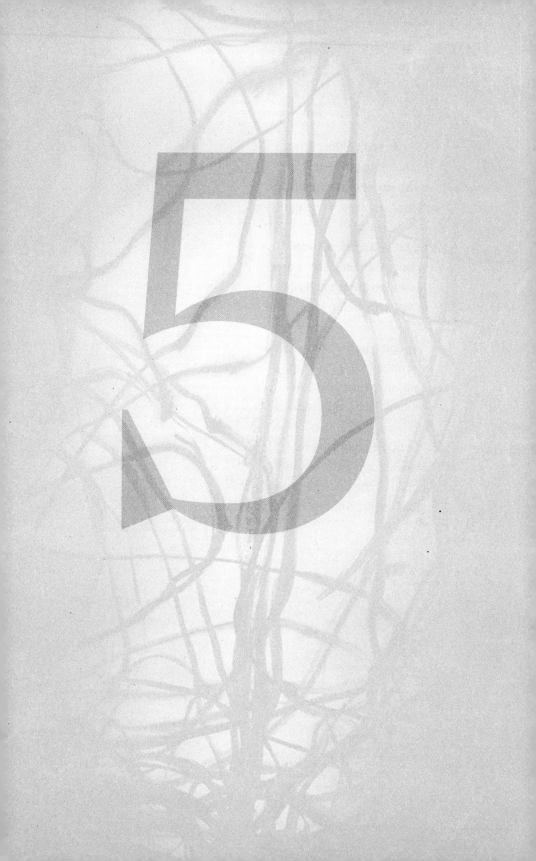

Apollo

We stepped on the surface
of the moon, strangers
tying scarves into blindfolds,
setting our feet in one direction

tentative, tottering cakes
of dust sketching salted arcs
in sand to the left and right
as we stepped out

one going back to her
starting place,
a misshapen circle,
ground flaked and cracking.

When they came to me,
I ran like a sentient arrow
pulled by the bow of my daughter
who saw me coming, caught my arm.

Fatu Hiva

I saw the end before I reached the top—
the vanishing tail
of a wide gravel road. Shade.

You had broken off at some point—
gone up ahead more quickly and left me
with two blondes, my halting French.

Unable to conjugate—verbs only for now
now I was cut off
like a Wernicke's aphasic

from connection, comprehension.
Waiting for you to reciprocate
my sacrifice. The trail kept getting steeper.

Ahead, your whole life was contained
within a question, your chest wall
and breast pocket burning

a fulcrum between past and present.
The trees thinned out. The heat
of the sun bore its full weight.

Alone, scaling a foreign mountain,
feet slipping on the scree.
At the top, you were waiting—

face full of concern, too late. I refused
to sit. To eat. Began my descent
not looking at you, at the vista.

Me, spitting with rage, you scrambling,
stepping sideways,
can we talk about this later?

Then, running ahead, you rounded a corner,
got down on one knee.
I found you like that as I came past

the switchback, framed by foliage,
sun glinting off the ocean.
The unexpressed now spoken.

Between Us

That week I didn't sleep,
husband gone and soother spit
up every forty-five minutes.
Came to the blunt end of myself

boundaries breached by a graphic
movie played on repeat
those first eight weeks she was home:
fontanelle, metal hairclip, levered arm

plunging. Had to use elastics.
Can still hear the clanging can
as the demon hit the garbage.
You couldn't be alone then, either,

near the window, in your bedroom
with your baby's bright face
screwed up, wailing eleven hours
a day for ten full months.

His soft skull hitting the pavement—
you could hear it. We were
the only mothers we knew
who dressed our babies roughly

and something passed between us:
you brought me Amish friendship
bread and ate on my deck.
Parts fitting together. We ate again

on murky banks of river Thames
and talked about what happens
when vaginas stay broken. Managed
to stay friends amidst watermelon

birthdays, you leaving your husband,
moving into my basement. I held you
as you wept—that night in the truck
out on the street—fourteen years pretending

you liked making laundry soap.
When you left, you crawled
across the dark on your knees.
Joy arrived in lost parts of yourself.

When a baby died as I attended,
halfway out
before his mother could hold him,
darkness fused to light.

I wandered the house
in a crocheted blanket—so wrecked,
you were a chasm away
in my yellow room

on a patterned chair across from
need I couldn't speak.
You reached for me,
came and laid down

on that small blue couch,
stroking my hair as I told you, sobbing,
what happened to that mother
and her baby—

what my hands had to do.
You didn't turn away.
We don't have a name for
what breathes between us.

Tried holding hands but it never felt
right—one of our palms twisted
an awkward direction,
so we melted instead and I slid

my wrist past the crook
of your elbow, intertwining arms,
heads dipping sideways,
feet falling into step.

The Bridge Between the Mountains

I took you with me
to the place of wind

where cicadas sang
and poetry was engraved

into sidewalks. Our steps
were lit like streetlamps

and there was space
big enough for big feelings

where mountains met
the ocean, met

my children's faces
as they looked out

and I saw them
as if for the first time,

saw time pouring through
us, saw them

in another life where I
did not have to sacrifice

them to save someone else.
I took you with me

as a testament, a witness
to the life I had chosen

and the chance I found
there, in that gap

between the mountains,
where sunshine burst

past the penumbra,
beyond its shadow revealing

the outline of a bridge
where I saw, I could cross.

I Have Passed Through

the Valley of Baca,
mud-caked and soaking,
leaves in my hair. You said

my voice was vitriolic.
Asked if I could
forgive, sincerely.

For the first time, I could
see myself biting
on the past; the past

was still biting
me: it was not you
anymore. A new choice:

set down this Ebenezer
stone of remembrance,
this golden pyramid

engraved on every side
by haunted loons.
As shadows lengthened

I set it down, I set it down
on autumn plains. Shorn.
Backlit and glinting,

I set it down, and set out,
carrying my sheaves
with me, rejoicing.

Lichen Sclerosis

is a tethering
of skin, an itching inflammation

pain fibres twitching
hand clawing compulsion

of bedroom excoriation,
scratching in the dark

since he left his mark
and the body said no

triggering confusion
of who the enemy is

leading to resorption—
my immune system turned

cannibalistic, eating
tender skin of my vulva

open, angry ulcers,
disfiguring the labia

sealing off clitoris.
In remission

I finally got angry.

The Stone the Builders Rejected

Burning and buried
for thirty-one years, I did not know
that felsic lava, cooled,
becomes a place of healing

and safety. Known as obsidian
black, it cracks like glass
and is used for tools—
sharp edges that slice

like a threshing blade.
When the shaman came,
wielding rock and
a smooth silver teapot

with two cups, she cut
the eschar than encased me.
Pink-skinned, marked
with skin grafts and scars

I set out on a quest
to offer the same,
and came upon a town
with a high central tower of bricks

housing a group of scientists
carrying the curse
of leprosy, faces wet
from open-roofed rain.

I laboured there for fourteen years,
but all the while I frightened them,
raw skin and stories
flayed open by love.

They did not listen or look
as I pointed to the tower,
crumbling, not made of ivory,
and they did not want

the black stone in my hand,
they did not feel,
nerve roots blunted,
so I left, taking my freedom with me

shaking the dust from my feet.
Obsidian black, once a trap,
once a stumbling block,
now the scalpel blade I work with.

Animal, Misunderstood

I said no when he asked me
but he made his case

saying he would pay
and feed and care for it.

Violent, I said
creepy, disgusting

I was sure till he pleaded—
they're misunderstood!

His compassion ignited
mine, and now a python

sleeps at his bedside.
Except when I notice

the empty terrarium,
and keep rifling,

holding my breath as I re-check
the layers of my bed sheets.

Wild Iris

I saw a wild iris on the boggy crags
of Tilting; *hard pressed on every side,*
but not crushed, delicate furling
purple sprung from rock and ice-
berg sunshine, *perplexed but not in despair.*
It persisted as the wind whipped
our faces, *struck down but not destroyed.*

Quiet, Rarely

I know the quiet

rarely, in moments:

indigo evening

when last light

finds a break

between branches

a figure of eight

hole of green

where leaves cast

their faces toward

my wicker chair

and insects hover,

dive into lavender,

the whippoorwill

calling to his brother.

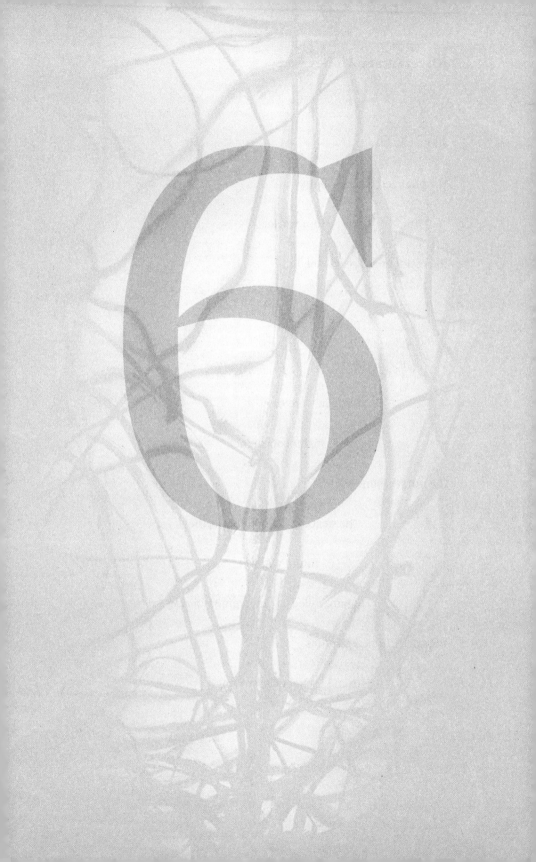

Alive. Intact. Unharmed.

1.

Hospitalized for back pain,

        thirty-four weeks,

the resident assessed you

     over-
         night: ruptured

membranes?

        But you were *fine*,

           just incontinent

the nurses wondered?

        The next day on the phone, they

          found you wet

        again, called   me, remembering

the sticky fifteen minutes

        in med school classroom

where grey hairs   taught

cauda equina

        ... she might

    never walk

2.

again, I ran—twisting

        a wooden tongue depressor

    into shards, said

        I have some awkward questions

 poked

    your inner thighs

      numb already

but couldn't actually

    prove or justify—

an experiment using dogs

    in the MRI machine.

        That happens?

3.

No time to clean it,

        delicate spinal

nerves dying by the minute

        horse's tail filaments

    crushed by

        lumbar bulge ballooning

    you're halfway

paralyzed

    I said
        I had to call
    neurosurg

        we've got a problem

and we flipped you like a pancake:

    one side for baby,
    one side for spine.

4.

That beginning

like unspooled tape:

reams of curling ribbon,

oil-black and glistening,

garbled in my body.

I can never go back

and listen;

just a felt sense,

the base beat

in my chest and the pull of

my bed where I never

slept.

5.

You came screaming   lightsandsirens

                feet hanging from   your groin.

         Cord compressed   no blood flowing

               to his head

   stuck

                   his body

            halfway born.

6.

My smooth white gloves

    cocoon his chest

limp   and small   and cold.

              Get two nurses   hold your thighs, push

                   push   to the walls   your knees

              you're scared *we know*

                     push push push—

7.

Make a fist   shove it   hard

      deep   deep

          into your pelvis

           flex   compress   dislodge

his head

    wasn't getting any oxygen

8.

     till   *pop—*

       and I pass his body

to waiting guard of yellow gowns

    armed with tubes and wires

       try, try,   try

    to get a heart rate.

9.

My mother asked me, late

in my training, *do you still look*

at the babies?

Acknowledgements

Thank you to the editors of the following publications where poems in *Python Love* previously appeared:

> *The Examined Life Journal* (US): "The Woman Beneath the Sheet,"
>   Fall 2020.
> *Snapdragon* (US): "Windless Sea" (previously "Defenseless"),
>   Fall 2021.
> *The Antigonish Review*: "Bed Rest Lament," Fall 2022.
> *PRISM International*: "Tidal Pools with my Mother,"
>   Summer 2023.
> *Contemporary Verse 2*: "Apollo," Summer 2024.

Thank you also to Anstruther Press, which published section 4 of this book as *Fallen Horseman* in 2023.

Python Love would not have been possible without the following people: Jim Johnstone, for his editorial support, kindness, and vision; Shane Nielson, for his keen eye and generous spirit; Ronna Bloom, for her coaching and mentorship at a stage when I didn't yet know what a poem was; Karen Wallace, for her wisdom and partnership at my darkest hours; my family, who saw me through all of it and loved me; and the cloud of witnesses who attended me with care, with tears, and with laughter. Thanks also to the writing group I participated in from 2021 to 2022, which included Shelley Harder, Kevin Heslop, Erica McKeen, Kit Roffey, and Jack Copeland—you were instrumental to everything that has happened since.